Downside of Nutrition part I

by Dr. Maxwell Nartey, DHM, NHD

RED LEAD PRESS
PITTSBURGH, PENNSYLVANIA 15222

The contents of this work including, but not limited to, the accuracy of events, people, and places depicted; opinions expressed; permission to use previously published materials included; and any advice given or actions advocated are solely the responsibility of the author, who assumes all liability for said work and indemnifies the publisher against any claims stemming from publication of the work.

Red Lead Press
701 Smithfield Street
Pittsburgh, PA 15222
Visit our website at *www.redleadbooks.com*

ISBN: 978-1-4349-6648-3
eISBN: 978-1-4349-2625-8

Downside of Nutrition
Part I

THIS BOOK IS AN INSIGHTFUL SCIENCE-BASED REVIEW OF THE foods we value. Also, it sounds a note of caution about health repercussions to those who are not careful in selecting the foods they eat and the beverages they consume. Certainly, it is a priceless treasure for every person who wants to take a proactive role in maintaining health.

CONTENTS

I dedicate this book to
Life, the greatest teacher that taught me a lot
through humility, observation and critical thinking

ACKNOWLEDGEMENTS

I remain profoundly indebted to my wife, Millicent, my son, Harold and my daughters: Adelrita, Isabella and Rosalita who used their talents, administrative and accounting skills to help me to launch symptometry, originator of root-cause therapeutics

INTRODUCTION

NUTRITION HAS TWO SIDES: A) AN UPSIDE THAT ONLY HIGHLIGHTS the nutrients in foods and in beverages and b) a downside where lay both nutrients and health disruptors. This book discusses the downside of nutrition that nutritionists have been avoiding like the plague.

Nutrition is the process of transferring tissue contents and molecules to the digestive system by eating and drinking. Nutrients are in the form of food, water, beverage and supplement molecules. A department of nutrition has been created in many universities and colleges to teach nutrition.

The purpose of teaching nutrition is not to teach people how to chew food and drink water or a beverage but rather how to use scientific research to enlighten the general public on the dietary habits that will help to eradicate diseases and promote health.

Deficiency diseases such as osteoporosis, scurvy, Paget's disease, etc. have been ruining health as far back as one can remember. However, it was the brilliant idea of one intuitive researcher after another that corrected the dietary mistakes that caused such diseases. This correction made people healthier. Let me cite a few examples.

People had been suffering from scurvy for thousands of years. Symptoms of scurvy include bleeding gums, wounds that won't heal and easy bruising. Nobody knew the cause of this disease.

In 1742, British physician James Lind linked scurvy to a dietary deficiency but he could not lay his finger on the missing nutrient. However, he recommended that people drink lemon juice or limejuice. The sailors who drank limejuice in 1804 did not have scurvy. Those who did not had the disease. It was not until 1928 that Albert Swent-Gyorgvi isolated vitamin C from limejuice to show that it was lack of vitamin C that caused scurvy.

In 1873, a Dutch naval doctor observed that the boat crew that were recruited from the East Indies suffered from beriberi more than the deck hands that were recruited from Europe. He could not figure out why this was happening. It was Dr. Takaki, a Japanese naval doctor who observed that the sailors who ate dry milk, vegetables and meat in addition to white rice did not suffer from beriberi. He then established that beriberi was caused by a certain nutrient deficiency.

In 1926, Jansen and Donath, two Dutch scientists, isolated thiamin from rice hull. This discovery was significant because it showed that the process of milling removed thiamin from rice. Then, it was eating rice, which lacked thiamin that caused beriberi. Governments then passed a law making the enrichment of white rice mandatory. Today, thanks to this nutritional research, nobody suffers from beriberi after eating white rice.

Since 1922, nutritional scientists had been aware of the role of vitamin A in the reproductive functions of humans as well in the retina. Also, in 1922, researchers discovered that rats, which were fed food that was deficient in vitamin E did not reproduce.

In China, researchers observed that most people from the Keshan province suffered from cancer and a kind of cardiovascular disease called Keshan disease. When the soil was tested it was found to be lacking selenium. After the provincial government passed a law making the incorporation of selenium into the soil mandatory, the cancer rate as well as the incidence of heart disease dropped significantly.

These are a few examples showcasing the contribution of scientific research to the promotion of health. My problem is there are people who drink limejuice and still bleed from their gums. I used to be one of them. Then, there are people who eat foods that are deficient in vitamin E and yet they are able to have children. People can eat foods that have selenium and yet they will have cancer; and people can eat foods that have vitamins and yet they will suffer from vitamin deficiency. This is the puzzle that nutritional research has not been able to solve.

The downside of nutrition is that it creates an illusion. The illusion it creates is the impression that eating a balanced diet and taking vitamins is the right way to prevent diseases. It is not.

A person can eat right and still suffer from hair loss. A woman can eat right and still have menstrual problems. A child can eat right and still feel tired most of the time.

There are over 3,000 ailments that eating vitamin-enriched and mineral-enriched foods will never help us to prevent or cure. Are these mysteries? No, they are not. It is nutritional research that has not gone far enough.

Symptometry is the field of applied therapeutic science that could be perceived as the natural extension of medical diagnostics, conventional medicine, homoeopathy, nutrition and naturopathy. It teaches what these above-listed disciplines don't teach. What don't departments of nutrition teach?

They don't teach root cause therapeutics. Implied in root cause therapeutics is disease prevention. Also, departments of nutrition don't teach that there are health disruptors in most fruits, legumes, vegetables, cooking oils and grains.

It is health disruptors that make people sick. How do they make people sick? It depends on the chemicals that the item, which was ingested releases into the body.

The chemicals and the acids that foods release into the body include cyanide, oxalic acid, prussic acid, salicylates, valeric acid and alkali. Processed foods have synthetic chemicals and these chemicals deplete B vitamins and chromium from the body.

Therefore, teaching that fruits and vegetables only supply fresh nutrients is inaccurate. Also, teaching that eggs, fish, seafood and meat supply only protein is very misleading.

All fishes and meats are not created equal. Most seafood feed on the heavy metals, wastes etc. that are on the riverbed or on the ocean floor. Since a person who eats seafood is transferring some of their tissue contents into h/her body, a person who eats fish that fed on heavy metals will also have some of these metals in h/her tissues.

A person who has health disruptors will never be healthy on all the seven fronts. A woman is not supposed to have vaginal discharge, she is not supposed to bleed between her periods, have menses for less than 4 to 5 days or for more than six days, have clots in her menstrual blood and so on and so forth.

Also, a child is not supposed to be irritable unless s/he is hungry. A man is not supposed to have an erection unnecessarily. Also, a person is not supposed to be angry for no reason or s/he is not supposed to be violent. It is health disruptors in the form of deficiencies and blockages that cause all these ailments.

A healthy person functions within the paradigm of normalcy. This paradigm governs our sexual behavior, mental attitude, emotional behavior, physical appearance, metabolic functions, and functions of our organs and circulatory system. This is why when a person's behavior is out of line those who are still within the paradigm of normalcy can sense it. They are feeling it because there was a deviation from the paradigm of normalcy.

Nobody imposed a code of behavior on us. The totality of our cells instinctively knows right from wrong. This is why they impart this knowledge to our mind.

Symptometry discovered that when cells are congested or they are deficient in certain nutrients they cause behaviors or symptoms that signal a deviation from normalcy. Since nutrition and conventional medicine cannot solve this problem at the cellular level, symptometry has to step in to provide root cause therapeutics.

This book draws the reader's attention to the health disruptors in the foods we love and to the dangers they pose to human lives. It also discusses the underlying cause of deficiency diseases so that the reader can take proactive measures to maintain health.

CHAPTER ONE
SCAVENGER FOODS AND NUTS

GOOD NUTRITION IS NOT A MATTER OF EATING WHAT IS AVAILABLE or what is culturally acceptable. Food must be selected very carefully so that our cells and our kidneys are not hurt after a meal.

Most seafood feed on heavy metals, wastes etc. that lie on the riverbed or on the ocean floor. This is why they are called scavengers.

Scavengers include: lobsters, crabs, shrimp, oysters, snails and crawfish. The shell of lobsters, crabs, crawfish and shrimp produce tough debris after metabolism. If the kidney cells cannot produce enzymes to liquefy this kind of debris, the kidneys will be jammed.

People can eat scavengers but it is the supplements they take after eating these foods that will help their cells to produce the enzymes that liquefy heavy metals and tough debris. If a person does not know the kinds of supplements to take, and the right time to take them, s/he may become susceptible to cancer or to kidney disease years after eating scavengers.

Nuts and seeds have minerals that our cells can use. Unfortunately, these minerals come at a price. This is because they are immersed in saturated fat or in salicylates. Our cells don't separate saturated fat from minerals. We will have to do the separation before we supply minerals to our cells.

All nuts have saturated fat and prussic acid. The fatty acid in saturated fat tends to slow down circulation. If this happens in the pores, acne will occur. Then, after the tough coat of the nut has been digested, it will produce tough debris. Saturated fat will slow down circulation; and slow circulation will cause stasis (circulatory disorder).

We can eat whatever we want but it is the supplements we take after eating certain foods that will help our cells to produce certain enzymes. Then, it is these enzymes that will neutralize the toxic effects of what we have eaten.

Plant enzymes are for the plant. They are not for humans. By the same token, animal hormones are for animals. They are not for humans.

In order to produce human enzymes and hormones, a person must decongest h/her cells and glands and s/he must supply the cells what they use to produce enzymes and hormones. If s/he doesn't, s/he will be deficient in testosterone, estrogen, progesterone, steroids and so on and so forth. Then, s/he will suffer from diseases associated with such deficiencies.

Chapter Two
Red Meat

THERE IS A DIFFERENCE BETWEEN RED MEAT FROM FREE-RANGE animals and red meat from sequestered animals. Sequestered animals that provide red meat include: cattle and hogs.

Sheep and goats don't make good sequestered animals. This is because they are antibiotic resistant and also, they easily succumb to cluster phobia.

Free-range cattle, sheep and goats do not have animal drugs in them but the sequestered ones do. Also, free-range cattle, sheep and goats have less saturated fat than the sequestered ones. A person who consumes beef from sequestered cattle will also ingest animal drugs and a lot of saturated fat. Lean beef has less saturated fat but it also has as many animal drugs as regular or whole meat.

The animal drug called sulfamethazine is found in beef, chicken, turkey and pork. It either predisposes a person to obesity or to fat accumulation in certain parts of h/her body. Then, it will reduce h/her resistance to diseases. Why is allergy on the rise? It is because sulfamethazine makes the cells of susceptible individuals to release a lot of histamines. Also, it makes the T cells less aggressive in the blood that has too much glucose.

Milk, lamb and goat meat have the highest amount of phenylalanine. Pregnant women who abstain from fish, meat, and goat meat or from lamb and who do not drink cow's milk risk giving birth to a child who will suffer from PKU (phenylketonuria).

Phenylalanine is an essential amino acid. This means our liver cannot produce it. It has to come from certain foods particularly goat meat, lamb and soymilk.

A vegetarian could get a small amount of it from soymilk but not from rice milk or from almond milk. All the thyroid hormones are produced from tyrosine. But the liver must have phenylalanine before it can produce tyrosine.

The brain uses about 70% of phenylalanine that we supply to our body. This is because it is the raw material from which norepinephrine is produced. However, in order to produce norepinephrine, the following nutrients must also be in the brain and adrenal cells: copper, vitamin C, pyridoxine, zinc and niacin.

Norepinephrine is the neurotransmitter that relaxes a person, it lowers blood pressure and it enhances memory activity, alertness and learning when too much glucose is not in blood.

Why are some people forgetful? Why are some students academically dull? Why do some people have a short attention span or they easily lose the focus of a discussion? The reason is they are not producing enough norepinephrine and acetylcholine. Hypertension is also common among individuals who are irritable or are forgetful. Lack of norepinephrine in a person who suffers from sugar imbalance is one of the factors that accounts for hypertension.

CHAPTER THREE
VEGETABLES

MOST FRUITS AND VEGETABLES SUPPLY ONLY BETWEEN 10 AND 25% of nutrients. The rest are chemicals such as oxalic acid, prussic acid, valeric acid, malic acid and cyanide that will disrupt our health by depleting B vitamins and chromium.

Do we eat to be healthy or we eat to be sick? It looks as if each time we eat we are compromising our health.

Children who refuse to eat vegetables are being put off by the vegetables' taste. To them, vegetables taste awful.

The second reason children don't like eating certain vegetables is these foods make them constipate, irritable, and forgetful. Children have a reason for rejecting vegetables. Unfortunately, parents don't listen to them.

Children don't like it when they talk back at their parents but sometimes, they can't help it. They are frustrated. Some of the foods they are served make them sick because they deplete their B vitamin and chromium. Then, if they eat to please their parents, they will suffer from the consequences of sugar imbalance.

We all produce calculi, calcareous deposits, gouty deposits and tophi. If B vitamins and chromium are not in a person's body, blockages will take their place in our nerve cells, bone cells, muscle cells and skin cells. This is how cellular congestion occurs.

Cells that are congested will suddenly produce an acute symptom. If the acute symptom is treated with a mismatch, it will become chronic. A mismatch is a therapeutic product that does not decongest the cell or nourish it. It only makes a person feel better by alleviating the severity of h/her symptoms.

Eating certain fruits and vegetables is a good idea but before eating them, certain supplements must be taken so that enzymes could be produced to liquefy their toxic effects.

Sickness results from not removing or from not neutralizing the plant chemicals that deplete B vitamins, zinc and chromium from the cells of the spinal cord, the brain, the joints, the eyes, the ears, the skin, the eyelids, the tongue etc.

There are 220 segments in the human body. It is the segment, which is congested or deprived of nutrients that will produce a symptom or an abnormality.

We may eat a balanced diet but this does not mean we will be healthy on all the seven fronts. For instance, a person could eat a balanced diet and yet s/he could have chronic migraine. Why does s/he have migraine? The reason is s/he ate foods that depleted B vitamins and zinc from h/her cerebral capillaries and brain tissue. Let me now discuss why plants have to produce more poisons than nutrients.

Plants have life just like humans do; and life is a gift of creation. Every piece of creation has cells; and every cell is imbued with super-intelligence; multiple powers, zest for life, self-protection and self-preservation.

Plants must produce harmful alkaloids, acids and poisons to protect themselves because they don't have legs to run away from their enemies as animals do; and also, they don't have guns and bombs to protect their territories as governments do.

The kinds of harmful chemicals they produce in order to protect themselves include: oxalic acid, salicylates, malic acid, solanine, prussic acid, cyanide, strychnine, poison ivy acid, retinoic acid, mandelic acid, brucine, pyridine, citronellol, chrysophenol and methylxantines.

Spinach has a large amount of oxalic acid. What does oxalic acid do? It depletes B vitamins to cause stenosis (narrowing of the blood vessels). Of all the blood vessels, our capillaries have the smallest diameter. If oxaluria further narrows this diameter, blood will simply stop flowing through the capillaries to certain bones, extremities, eyes, ear, heart tissues, lung tissues etc.

Should myocardial infarction, dim vision and ringing in the ear or ischemia (bloodlessness) be a mystery? No, they should not. Stenosis causes them.

Oxaluria causes other ailments such as blue nails, brittle nails, black acne spots, carotenosis, chronic diarrhea and glaucoma.

In light of the above, I recommend that spinach be eaten only once or twice a week and B vitamins be taken after eating it.

Other legumes and vegetables that produce oxalic acid are: aramanth, asparagus, beet leaves, Brussels sprouts, carrots, cabbage, cauliflower, celery, chicory, collards, chives, egg plant, garlic, lettuce of all kinds, parsley, radishes, turnip and watercress.

If after eating a vegetable some of the above-listed symptoms occur, I recommend steering clear of that vegetable in the future or taking B vitamins and chromium to restore sugar balance.

CHAPTER FOUR
MILK

WHENEVER NUTRITIONISTS TALK ABOUT MILK WHAT THEY GEN-ERALLY say is it supplies calcium. Regrettably, calcium is not the only mineral in milk.

Even though dairy milk and non-dairy milk have calcium, phosphorus, magnesium and sulfur, there is a significant difference between dairy and non-dairy milk. Also, there is a difference between dairy milk from free-range goats and cattle; and dairy milk from sequestered cattle.

Dairy milk from sequestered cattle has animal drug residues. For instance, sulfamethazine and tylosin are in milk that was extracted from sequestered cattle. Secondly, the milk from sequestered cattle has saturated fat. This is the direct result of the growth hormone that was injected into them. Sulfamethazine predisposes a person to allergies, to fatty liver, fatty heart and to a weak immune system.

Cow's milk is not snow white. It was bleached with benzoyl peroxide, an allergen. Therefore, it is not cow's milk that causes sinusitis. It is benzoyl peroxide that predisposes a person to allergies and to sinusitis. This is because it makes the cells to over-produce histamine as it is depleting prostaglandin.

Cow's milk also has ammonium caseinate and traces of other animal drugs such as sulfaquinoxaline, procaine penicillin, profluralin, agribon, prednisdone, amoxillin trihydrate etc.

Sulfaquinoxaline causes photophobia and allergic reactions. Overplaying the importance of calcium, phosphorus etc. in cow's milk tends to make people to overlook the acidity of this milk as well as the sulfa drugs it has. Cow's milk is very acidic.

Sulfaethoxypiridazine is the antibiotic that is routinely added to the cattle's drinking water. In breast milk, the calcium phosphorus ratio is 2:1. In cow's milk, the calcium phosphorus ratio is 1:2. This is why, technically speaking, cow's milk cannot replace breast milk. A baby must have breast milk. If s/he can't, s/he could suffer from a few enzymatic disorders in the future.

Prednisone is chemically related to cortisol that is used to treat inflammations, ulcerative colitis and prostatitis. It depletes B vitamins, zinc and chromium to cause adverse reactions such as insomnia, euphoria, psychotic behavior, obesity, acid reflux, chronic belching, high blood pressure, swelling, cataract, glaucoma, peptic ulcer, diabetes mellitus, delayed wound healing, pancreatitis, decreased immunity and adrenal gland insufficiency.

People who drink cow's milk or eat beef that has a higher concentration of prednisone residues could experience some of the above-listed symptoms or medical conditions.

Baby formula is made from whey. Whey is the protein that is obtained by separating the watery part of cow's milk from curds. It becomes very acidic after two hours. If a baby is fed milk that was left standing in the bottle for more than two hours, s/he could develop acidosis, colic or diarrhea.

Most baby formulas have been enriched with DHA (docosahexaeonic acid) but not with EPA (eicosapentaeonic acid) and with GLA (gamma linolenic acid). These three oil chemicals are in breast milk. Since two of them are not in many baby formulas, inadequate oil-derived carbon will create an imbalance that will cause cell impermeability. Then, cell impermeability will cause dry skin in the baby.

Non-dairy milk includes plant milk such as: soymilk, almond milk, cashew milk, hemp milk and rice milk. Of all the non-dairy milks, soymilk has the highest amount of phenylalanine in addition to calcium, sulfur, phosphorus, magnesium and unsaturated fat. Rice milk has all the minerals that soymilk has except phenylalanine. Unfortunately, a person who cannot produce enzymes to break down genistein in soymilk could become allergic to soymilk or could have serious hormonal disorders.

The lower the calcium percentage in soymilk the better it will be for a person who has hypertension. Then, the higher the calcium percentage, the better soymilk or rice milk will be for a person who suffers from low blood pressure.

Compared to bottle milk, breast milk is healthier for the baby. This is because it has the right amount of fats, water, nutrients and white blood cells.

Most nursing mothers cannot breastfeed their baby because either they are not producing breast milk or they have milk in their breast but it won't flow. B vitamin deficiency accounts for this problem.

CHAPTER FIVE
SALICYLATES

A SALICYLATE IS AN ANION OF SALICYLIC ACID. AN ANION CARRIES a negative charge because it is releasing a lot of electrons. Most of our cells don't need too many electrons in their nuclei. This is why a surplus of electrons will create electron imbalance in the body.

Chromium is very sensitive to electron imbalance. Lack of chromium will translate to sugar imbalance. Then, sugar imbalance will interfere with the vagus nerve's ability to receive and transmit signals to the carotid cells in the brain. Signal interference could result in low blood pressure, seizure or in hypertension.

People react to electron imbalance differently. In some individuals, it could cause hypertension. In others, it could cause excessive belching, chronic fatigue, seizure, and bloating or gassiness. Foods that have salicylates include:

- Almonds
- Apples
- Apple cider
- Apricot
- All berries
- All cherries
- Cucumbers
- Cloves
- Currants
- Grapes
- Nectarines
- Oranges

- Pickles
- Peaches
- Plums
- Prunes
- Raisins and
- Raw tomato

My advice has always been, watch what you eat. If after eating a fruit or a vegetable blood pressure rises, and belching or bloating occurs, the food that was eaten is causing electron imbalance. Consult a symptometrist to correct this imbalance.

CHAPTER SIX
CHICKEN EGGS

BASICALLY, AN EGG HAS TWO COMPONENTS: A) YOLK AND b) albumin (egg white). Yolk has a large amount of animal cholesterol in addition to oil, sulfur and other nutrients. Albumin is very alkaline. Its pH is 8.5 whereas the pH of blood is 7.4.

The animal drugs that are in the eggs of sequestered poultry include: sulfamethazine and tylosin. Both will slow down a person's metabolism. Then, there is salmonella in all eggs.

The skin is acidic because its pH (acid/alkaline ratio) is around 6.0. If the skin absorbs the alkalinity of albumin, a susceptible person could suffer from eczema, weird skin disorder, and dry skin or hives.

Eczema is another form of dermatitis (inflammation of the skin). People who are allergic to eggs could suffer from eczema after eating eggs. In the worse case scenario, albumin could cause anaphylaxis. Many vaccines are cultured in albumin. A person who is susceptible to albumin could suffer a severe reaction after a vaccination.

Egg powder is in many shampoos, ointments and creams. The reason for adding egg powder to these cosmetics is that sulfur is beneficial to the damaged hair or damaged skin. This theory is not scientifically tenable because many women tend to lose their hair after using certain shampoos.

Also, certain creams, lotions and ointments tend to inflict more damage on the skin. Facial mask is made from albumin. If the concentration of albumin in the facial is too high, it could damage the skin's cross-links. As a result, wrinkles could start appearing very early.

13

There is egg in ice cream, doughnut, mayonnaise, cake etc. There are many particulates that will decongest the cells in order to cure eczema, hives etc. However, if the person who is being treated continues to eat foods that have eggs, there could be a relapse.

Some people crave eggs. Usually, such individuals are not healthy because consuming a highly alkaline food amounts to self-destructive behavior. Eating raw egg introduces salmonella typhi to the gastrointestinal tract. The presence of this bacterium will cause food poisoning, typhoid or salmonellosis. Because of the constant presence of salmonella in raw eggs, eggs should be handled with great care.

CHAPTER SEVEN
FRUITS

MOST FRUITS ARE NOT AS HARMLESS AS NUTRITIONISTS CLAIM.
The fruits that are harmless are: watermelon (but not for people who are
overweight or suffer from edema), pineapple, ripe banana (not for diabet-
ics), avocado and ripe guava (the juice is preferable). The rest of the fruits
could be very harmful to the central nervous system as well as to the periph-
eral nervous system. How do fruits harm the nervous system?

There is an enzyme in every synaptic cleft. Then, there is also acetylcholine in many clefts. The purpose of the enzyme is to speed up signal transmission and reception so that the impulse that a nerve transmits is received
in one tenth of a second by the dendrites.

Citronellol and citric acid that are found in all citrus fruits will denature
this enzyme. Citrus fruits include: lemon, lime, clementine, grapefruit,
kumquart, mandarin, Minneola, orange, pummelo, Satsuma, sweety, tan-
gerine, tangelo and Ugli.

A denatured enzyme will slow down signal transmission to the point
where a person could become forgetful or s/he could experience irritability,
numbness, cramps or spasms. Pain is associated with cramps.

Additionally, citric acid from the above-listed fruits will chelate calcium
ions. To chelate means to tie up the ions of a specific mineral so that the mineral in question does not get into the cells or tissues. It is a kind of blockade.
Chelation is very popular in chemotherapy because it prevents metals in
drugs from flooding the patient's body during cancer treatment.

Why are so many people suffering from calcium deficiency diseases such as brittle bones, dental cavities, sensitive teeth, soft bones, weak spinal cord, bone pain, etc? It is not because they are eating the wrong foods.

Basically, every food has calcium. This is because calcium is required for cell division in plants as well as in animals. It is concentrated citric acid that prevents calcium from getting into a person's cells. This is how citrus fruits cause calcium deficiency.

Malic acid is in apples, strawberries and in grapes as well as in cherries. It causes fatigue, lack of focus and hyperactivity.

Focusing only on the nutrients that fruits have amounts to discussing a half-truth. Malic acid does exactly what citronellol does to the nervous system. All type A personalities are suffering from B vitamin deficiency as well as from the effects of denatured enzymes in their synaptic clefts.

Because of the damage that fruit acids do to the nervous system, I recommend that acid fruits be eaten only between 11 a.m. and 3 p.m. This gives the pancreas enough time to rest.

A well-rested pancreas will harness enough resources to produce high-quality pancreatic enzymes for the morning and evening meals. Also, if a person takes B vitamins about 45 minutes after a meal, s/he will help h/her cells to produce replacement enzymes as quickly as possible.

Eating acid fruits at the wrong time (morning and evening) will compel the pancreas to produce low-quality enzymes for digestion. An overworked pancreas could become inflamed (pancreatitis) or it could become cancerous especially if blockages are preventing oxygen from getting into the pancreatic cells.

Banana is an acid fruit. But its amyl acetate (banana oil) prevents its hydrogen ions from denaturing the enzymes in the body. Secondly, it is the best source of soluble fiber. Women who lack soluble fiber may end up suffering from fibroid tumors. The colons need a lot of soluble fiber everyday in order to enhance peristalsis (wavelike movement) and promote regular bowel movement.

Unfortunately, a person who suffers from acid reflux or from diabetes mellitus will be worse off after eating banana. This is why, even though banana is an excellent fruit, I won't recommend it to a diabetic or to a person who suffers from heartburn.

Chapter Eight

Cyanide

A FEW PLANTS PROTECT THEMSELVES WITH CYANIDE. THEY absorb a lot of nitrogen from the soil. Then, they combine it with different acids in order to produce a potent poison called cyanide.

Plants that have cyanide include:

- Corn and all its derivatives (corn oil, corn syrup, etc.)

- Flax and flaxseed/linseed

- Apricot

- Cherries

- Peach

- Plums

- Lima bean

Cyanide is harmful because it is a pentose eliminator. We all have DNA in our cells. DNA consists of a) phosphoric acid b) amino acids and c) pentose that is also called ribose.

Pentose is the five-carbon sugar that serves as the backbone of DNA. If it is eliminated, DNA will collapse in less than one minute. Then, it will turn into uric acid; and uric acid will turn into gout. In other words, people who regularly consume foods that have cyanide will suffer from frequent gout attacks. Pain is associated with gout. Cyanide will also deplete zinc from the body. Natural painkillers and melatonin for sleep can't be produced without zinc

Furthermore, cyanide will deplete B vitamins and chromium. This explains why people who eat foods that have cyanide tend to suffer from diseases or symptoms caused by sugar imbalance such as hypoglycemia, diabetes mellitus, criminal intent and behavior, violent temper, irritability, etc.

In light of the above, it is recommended that people who eat corn, lima bean, etc. should take zinc, chromium and B vitamins the next day. Foods don't supply these nutrients in their concentrated form.

CHAPTER NINE
TEA

TANNIC ACID AND PALMITIC ACID TURN TEA INTO AN ACID BEVERAGE. Its catechins are iron inhibitors and its palmitic acid will block osmosis. Blockage of osmosis in the gallbladder could cause the formation of gallstones. In the bladder, such a blockage will cause the depletion of pyridoxine. In the absence of pyridoxine, bladder stones will form in the bladder and kidney stones will form in the kidneys.

Blockage of osmosis and the depletion of pyridoxine can also cause kidney problems such as acute nephritis, nephritis or glomerulonephritis (Bright's disease).

Even though both have methylxanthines, tea and coffee are two different plants. Cocoa and coffee have theobromine. Tea does not have theobromine. It has theophylline.

Theobromine is a diuretic, a vasodilator and a smooth muscle relaxant. In other words, a person who drinks or who eats cocoa products or drinks coffee, will experience frequent urination. Then, h/her blood pressure will be temporarily low because theobromine is dilating h/her arteries.

The downside of theobromine is that it saturates the cells very quickly and this is what causes toxicity. Theobromine toxicity causes muscle spasms, insomnia, hilarity, diarrhea or nausea. In the worse case scenario, it could cause coma after head trauma.

On the other hand, theophylline in tea is a central nervous system stimulant, a bronchodilator and a cardiac muscle stimulant. This is why it is effective in minimizing the severity of asthma, emphysema, pulmonary obstruction, dyspnea (shortness of breath) and bronchitis.

Contrary to what people think, drinking tea does not raise a person's energy level. It only makes a person more alert for a brief period. This is because theophylline in tea is not the substitute for B vitamins and acetylcholine. It only mimics the way acetylcholine stimulates the central nervous system.

Tealeaves come from the evergreen plant of the camellia family (camellia sinensis). There is black tea, green tea and oolong tea. The different chemical properties that a category of tea has depend on how it was processed.

Tealeaves that were warmed for a few hours, were then heated up to 200 degrees Fahrenheit and were dried will become known as Black tea. Tealeaves that were just steamed will become known as green tea. Tealeaves that were heated at a temperature below 200 degrees Fahrenheit for a very short time will become known as oolong tea.

In order to differentiate one brand of tea from another, tea makers add certain preservatives or flavoring additives. This is why the tealeaves that are plugged from the tea farms in India, Sri Lanka, Ceylon, and China, etc. are not the same as those that are sold in supermarkets throughout the world.

For instance, green tea that is freshly plugged from a tea farm in China, Ceylon, Bangladesh, etc. is not the same as green tea that was packaged and shipped to Great Britain, the United States, France, etc. One is fresh from the farm without any synthetic chemicals and the other has been chemically processed and preserved for long shelf life.

Therefore, people who want to benefit from drinking fresh green tea should go to China, Sri Lanka, Thailand, and Ceylon or Bangladesh.

If a country's climate is not conducive to tea cultivation, the only way to get tea into that country is through importation. There are preservatives in imported tea, regular or decaffeinated.

CHAPTER TEN
COFFEE

TANNIC ACID AND PALMITIC ACID TURN COFFEE AND COCOA INTO an acid beverage and substance. Both cocoa and coffee have theobromine, a form of methylxanthine.

Theobromine will combine with pyridine to block the diffusion of nutrients into the pleasure centers of the brain. Then, as non-nutrients, they will take over the process of cell division in the pleasure centers. The take over will cause coffee receptors to mushroom in the pleasure centers. Then, it is the presence coffee receptors in the hippocampus that will cause coffee addiction in the regular coffee drinker.

The difference between regular and decaffeinated coffee lies in the amount of theobromine in the beverage. Decaffeinated coffee has less theobromine than regular coffee. This is why it will take several years of drinking decaffeinated coffee on a daily basis to transform a regular "decaf" drinker into a coffee addict.

Theobromine depletes B vitamins especially pantothenic acid that is very important for hydrolysis in the mitochondria. Without hydrolysis, cells will not be able to produce enough energy. This will cause exhaustion, lethargy or chronic fatigue.

Tough debris that forms in the pineal gland in the absence of B vitamins will prevent the production of melatonin for sleep. This will cause insomnia or un-refreshing sleep in the coffee drinker.

Furthermore, coffee filters contain dioxin; and dioxin is a cancer-causing agent because it depletes oxidase. Without oxidase many cells will not be able to get and use oxygen. How do coffee drinkers get cancer? It could come from dioxin.

Health is an individual effort to return the cells to their state of perfection. A person can drink tea and coffee but if s/he knows the supplements that s/he will have to take after drinking these beverages, s/he will never suffer from theobromine toxicity.

Many homoeopathic particulates may lose their efficacy if a person who takes them also drinks coffee.

A person who has mastered the overriding technique can drink whatever s/he wants and s/he will still be healthier than a person who abstains from all kinds of foods and beverages for health reasons.

The comedian George Burns, smoked cigar for more than 75 years. There is tobacco in cigar. Tobacco causes cancer because it's carbon monoxide depletes oxygen and oxidase.

George Burns died at age 100 (January 20, 1896 – March 9, 1996) without ever being diagnosed with cancer. Therefore, what is most important in health is the awareness about what to do after smoking, after drinking or after eating items that have health disruptors.

Chapter Eleven
Purines

Purine is a component of nucleic acids (DNA and RNA). When a person eats foods that eliminate purine, s/he should know the foods that are its richest source so that s/he can eat them. This will help to replace what was depleted. Important purines are uric acid, adenine, xanthines and guanine.

We are always eliminating uric acid with urine. In order to minimize the elimination of uric acid, we can supply our body purines by eating anchovies, mushrooms, sardines, asparagus and organ meats especially the liver. But here too, there is a catch.

The liver is a poison processor. Since the condition of the animal was not known before it was slaughtered, eating animal liver could be risky.

Coffee has methylxanthines. This is why it is an excellent purine stimulant especially in the central nervous system. Unfortunately, pyridine, theobromine, palmitic acid and theophelline will abort such stimulation after two to three hours. The reason is that pyridine, theobromine and theophelline are not real B vitamins. They just mimic how B vitamins work.

Usually, a coffee drinker loses energy and alertness after two to three hours. This is because the pretenders don't supply the cells what they need in order to produce enzymes for the synaptic cleft.

Mushrooms have succinic acid and sterols. The demerits of succinic acid as an enzyme destroyer far outweigh the merits of purine and sterols that mushrooms have. Whatever mushrooms have, are for the mushrooms. They are not for humans.

Why is it that antibiotics and cholesterol-lowering drugs that are made from mushrooms have awful side effects? The reason is our cells don't need them. Our cells will produce their own cholesterol, hydrogen peroxide and bacteriocin if we supply them the right raw materials.

Sardines, anchovies and asparagus do not have health disruptors but a person who cannot produce enzymes to thoroughly digest their protein may have a skin disorder after eating them.

Foods that supply the lowest amount of purines include: bread, cereals, fats, cheese, eggs, fruits, milk and nuts.

Therefore, if we want to rebuild DNA and for that matter the genes, we will have to eat foods that are the richest source of purine. Then, we should also get cobalt from vitamin B12.

Chapter Twelve
Vanadium

There are 115 known minerals. Out of this number, only 26 are in human tissues. Vanadium is not one of the 26. This means vanadium is not supposed to be in human tissues. It could be useful to a plant but not to a person. If vanadium does not play a role in human cells then, it will become a nutrient blocker.

Many herbalists tout the virtues of garlic as an all-purpose rhizome. They claim it lowers cholesterol and it has antibiotic properties. My question is can a person who is suffering from HIV/AIDS take garlic and h/her infection will be cured? Can a person who has elevated cholesterol take garlic and h/her LDL (bad cholesterol) will be lowered?

During my early years of practice, I recommended garlic to treat infectious mononucleosis and high LDL. It failed miserably. I had an in-law who was fond of eating garlic everyday. He developed a tumor in his palate. As a result, he died a horrible death.

I personally do not see how a person who consumes a nutrient blocker will be healthy. Our cells need all the nutrients they can get. Sugar imbalance is already blocking many nutrients from diffusing into our cells. Why consume a food item that has a nutrient blocker, especially vanadium?

The items that have vanadium include:

- Olive oil; heating it will soften its vanadium

- Garlic

- Corn

- Buckwheat

- Parsley

- Soybean

- Safflower oil

- Raw onions

- Oats

- Sunflower seeds

- Green beans

- Peanut oil

- Carrots

- Cabbage (raw and cooked)

- Raw tomato

- Whole wheat

- Radishes

- Beets

- Apples

- Plums

- Lettuce of all kinds

- Millet

With the exception of olive oil and onions whose vanadium will be softened after heating them for 5 minutes, the vanadium in all the rest will remain what they are i.e. nutrient blockers. In other words, cooking them won't make a difference.

Also, there has been a lot of folklore about onions. One observation I have made is people who have tumors and men who have a high PSA (prostate specific antigen) are frequent consumers of garlic or raw onion. This means there is a correlation between the nutrient blocker in these items and the occurrence of a tumor. No wonder many experts consider garlic and raw onion to be first-class tumorigens.

A 60–year old man sought my expertise because his PSA was 43 (normal PSA is around 3.5). I asked him to list what he eats very often, almost on a daily basis. He mentioned onion. I asked him to explain why he liked eating raw onion so much? He told me onion is his sleep aid. Without it, he would be awake all night.

I asked him to refrain from eating onions. I decongested the cells of his prostate and brain and I nourished them. Then, I restored his sugar balance. He had been sleeping soundly ever since. After three months of treatment his PSA reading was 3.5. Not only was he very happy. He also began to warn people against eating raw onions, citing his own experience as an example.

Culture is responsible for total health-related ignorance in communities. Onion has to be cooked at all times. Adding sliced onion to hotdog or to salad is very unhealthy.

A popular folklore touts the antiviral properties of raw onions. It is said that onions attract viruses like a magnet and then, they destroy the viruses. This is why, according to folklore, if a person who has influenza or wants to prevent it places sliced onions in a plate and leaves it in h/her room, s/he will be cured or s/he will not have the disease.

One thing with me is I never dismiss folklore outright. I always try to understand the science behind every theory or folklore before I put it the test. If it fails or it passes the test, I will have a scientific explanation for its success or failure.

Onion has a lot of allyl sulfide. This is a sulfur compound that rearranges the isotopes of heat-damaged nutrients in order to revitalize them. For instance, the process of cooking damages many amino acids and vitamins. If onion is added to rice as it is boiling, the level of methionine will rise. Also, if onion is added to stew on the fire, it will reconstruct many nutrients whose isotopes were disorganized by intense heat.

Chicken soup that is prepared with onion is very effective against influenza and cold viruses. This is because intense heat softens vanadium in onion. Then, it unlocks phosphorus, calcium, folic acid and sulfur. The tattered cells will use these nutrients to repair themselves and healing will occur.

Once cell division resumes thanks to the presence of folic acid and calcium, the microtubules on which the viruses were hanging to transmit their DNA or RNA to the victim's cells will be wiped out. Without a foothold, viruses will disintegrate. This is how chicken soup that was prepared with onions is effective in providing temporary relief against viral infection of the upper respiratory tract.

Our grandmothers knew how to use chicken soup to treat the cold but they could not provide a scientific explanation for what they did. Raw onion in a plate could be effective against viruses in a room but what happens when a person is required by circumstances to leave h/her room for 10 hours? Won't s/he be vulnerable? Yes, s/he will.

Olive oil has vanadium but canola oil does not. This makes canola oil far better than olive oil on salad. Stew that was cooked with either canola oil or olive oil produces fewer lipid peroxides (blood vessel destroyers).

The betaglucans in oats bind with cholesterol in order to pull some of it out of the system. Unfortunately, oat has vanadium, which will block other nutrients from getting into the cells. Oat also has insoluble fiber. Insoluble fiber depletes zinc from the body. Without zinc, a person's pain threshold will be very low.

Lettuce regardless of its kind has many nutrients. Unfortunately, it also has vanadium that will block the diffusion of nutrients into the cells. Then, the insecticides in non-organic lettuce could make this vegetable a health hazard.

There is vanadium in millet, carrots, cabbage, green beans, etc. With the exception of cooked onions and heated olive oil whose vanadium has been softened by heat, I won't recommend foods whose vanadium cannot be softened.

Also, I won't recommend eating raw carrots. Every person that I treated and cured of glaucoma ate raw carrots. Vanadium will block the canal of schlemm and prevent the eye from draining its lymph. It is this blockage that will increase eye pressure and cause severe pain in the eye.

CHAPTER THIRTEEN
MOLYBDENUM

MOLYBDENUM IS NOT LISTED AMONG THE 26 MINERALS IN HUMAN tissue. This means it is supposed to be in plants but not in humans. If it is not supposed to be in humans then, in human tissue, it will be a nutrient blocker.

The items that have molybdenum include:

• Certain multivitamins

• Butter

• Corn

• Lentils

• Split peas

• Green peas

• Green beans

• Cauliflower

• Brewer's yeast

• Wheat germ

• Spinach

- Brown rice

- Garlic

- Oats

- Rye bread

- Barley

- Whole wheat

- Whole wheat bread

- Potatoes

- Onions

- Peanuts

- Cantaloupe

- Molasses

- Brown sugar

- Apricot

- Raisins

- Strawberries

- Carrots and

- Cabbage

Unlike vanadium in olive oil and onion that can be softened, heat cannot soften molybdenum in any plant.

A person who does not feel well after eating any of the above should immediately draw a connection between the nutrient blocker s/he consumed and the ailment. The body will react when it is not getting the nutrients it needs. This is because a blocking agent is in the system.

Chapter Fourteen
Brown Sugar, White Sugar

BROWN SUGAR IS MADE FROM MOLASSES. THIS MEANS IT HAS molybdenum that human cells don't need. If cells don't need a mineral and that mineral is still in the system, it could cause hyperplasia, a medical term for enlargement. In other words, it will cause tissue to stretch beyond its natural limit.

Examples of hyperplasia include: endometriosis where the tissue of the endometrium will spread to the vagina or to the brain; enlarged heart, enlarged liver, enlarged spleen and enlarged prostate.

White sugar is not made of only sucrose. Sucrose constitutes only one tenth of the sweetener called table sugar. The rest are additives including ammonium phosphate, a purifying agent.

Ammonium phosphate is a diuretic (causes frequent urination). After extracting sugar from sugar cane, sugar undergoes several chemical processes before it is sold to consumers as white sugar.

One of the final clarifying agents that are used to give sugar its final form is the preservative called aluminum potassium phosphate. It is insoluble in the human body. Any agent that is insoluble will be a nutrient blocker. Sugar is bleached with aluminum sodium sulfate. This chemical may cause skin rash.

Is it because of these demerits that sugar should not be eaten? A person has to consume sugar or the good sources of purines (see chapter eleven). This is because ribose/pentose, the five-carbon sugar that forms the backbone of DNA is made from sugar or from purines. Stevia is also another source of purines.

A person is a sugar-dependent being. This is why a person who does not eat sugar in moderation will suffer from the consequences of inadequate glucose. The most common symptom of inadequate glucose is irritability without cause.

Contrary to popular belief, eating sugar does not cause diabetes mellitus. It is a person's inability to produce sucrase, insulin, cortisol and liver enzymes that makes h/her susceptible to diabetes mellitus. Corn eaters are the frequent casualties of diabetes mellitus.

Chapter Fifteen
Brown Bread, White Bread

BROWN BREAD AND WHITE BREAD ARE MADE FROM WHEAT. THE difference is that brown bread is made from the testa (coat) of wheat and white bread is made from the endosperm, the equivalent of yolk.

The endosperm has all the nourishing nutrients for the wheat's growth and development whereas the testa only has the roughage that consists of insoluble fiber, cadmium, molybdenum and vanadium. Mother Nature uses these minerals to make the testa waterproof, insect proof and bird proof. Without this protection, water would have destroyed wheat, and birds and insects would have fed on wheat to create famine.

Brown bread, because of its high content of molybdenum, cadmium and vanadium, is mostly made of insoluble fiber. Humans need soluble fiber and not insoluble fiber. Insoluble fiber depletes zinc from the body. A person who does not have zinc will suffer from all kinds of inflammations including sarcoidosis.

Insoluble fiber causes incontinence and chronic constipation and sometimes, irritable bowel syndrome. Soluble fiber, that banana has helps the colons to produce elastin. This is more consistent with the needs of the bowels. It is for these contrasting reasons that I recommend eating white bread.

Unfortunately, all white breads are not created equal. "Sitting ducks" are the white breads that remain on the store shelves for more than 5 days. Since white bread becomes very acidic after three days, I recommend buying freshly baked white bread. Bread that has become acidic is just as harmful as citrus fruits or they are as harmful as the fruits that have malic acid (see page28).

Baking powder has tartaric acid; and flour must have aluminum potassium sulfate so that it does not cake. Most people who don't decongest their cells may find it difficult to digest bread for the reasons that are given below.

Aluminum potassium sulfate and calcium carbonate in bread will prevent the cells of the colons and throat from producing elastin. This will cause constipation or difficulty swallowing.

Bread has calcium bromate. This is a dough conditioner and a maturing additive that is added to bromate flour. Calcium bromate could cause difficulty breathing.

Then, flour is bleached with benzoyl peroxide. This chemical could cause constipation. Certain breads have ammonium chloride, a dough conditioner, or ammonium phosphate a leavening additive. Ammonium causes the kind of debris that only ammonium particulates can neutralize. These particulates are in the homoeopathic materia medica.

If eating bread causes stomach distress, I will suggest switching to eating waffles. Foods that were prepared with a very small amount of bromate flour or with flour that doesn't have calcium bromate don't cause bowel and stomach distress.

CHAPTER SIXTEEN
POULTRY

INCLUDED IN THE POULTRY CATEGORY ARE: GUINEA FOWL, CHICKENS, turkey and ostrich. Guinea fowl has the smallest amount of saturated fat in its tissue.

Free-range chickens are virus reservoirs. However, cooking them will kill all the viruses and make them safe to eat. Secondly, free-range chickens have less fat compared to sequestered chickens. Drugged chickens are unhealthy because they have animal drugs in their tissue.

Animal drugs such as chlortetracycline, sulfamethazine, sulfanitran and sulfadimethoxine will escape through the pores of the person who eats drugged animal. This may cause an offensive body odor or bad breath if s/he can't produce enzymes to break them down and liquefy them.

Chlortetracycline fattens chicken. Therefore, a person who eats drugged chicken is not only consuming flesh. S/he is also ingesting animal drugs and food additives. This could make h/her susceptible to obesity or to fatty liver or even to fatty heart. I recommend cooking skinless free-range chicken. This is because almost all the fats are concentrated in the chicken's skin.

Chlortetracycline makes antibiotics and anti-virals ineffective. Countless people are suffering from chronic gonorrhea or herpes because they eat chicken or beef that were treated with chlortetracycline. Chlortetracycline also makes methillin ineffective in the treatment of staphylococcus infection. Is HIV/AIDS incurable? It is curable. It is chlortetracycline and other antibiotics that make HIV/AIDS incurable.

MRSA (methillin resistant staphylococcus infection) occurs only in beefeaters and in individuals who eat drugged chicken. Flesh-eating bacteria (staphylococcus aureus) are active only on the flesh of individuals whose skin has retained traces of chlortetracycline.

Sulfomyxin that is a chicken antibiotic can cause photophobia and allergies. Other antibiotics are: sulfanitran, sulfaquinoxaline, sulfamethazine and streptomycin. Read more about streptomycin in the next paragraph. Spectinomycin that is also called stanilo is a chicken antibiotic. It causes hives, decreased urine output and chills. It is also a drug that is used to treat syphilis.

Sulfomyxin that is a turkey antibiotic could cause photophobia and allergic reactions. Other turkey antibiotics are sulfanitran, sulfaquinoxaline, sulfamethazine and streptomycin. Streptomycin has been implicated in aplastic anemia, muscle problems, kidney dysfunction, pain and skin disorders.

Weak heart and heart disease are common in individuals who were treated with streptomycin or who ate chickens and turkey that were drugged with streptomycin.

Chapter Seventeen
Pork

The meat of swine or hog is called pork. Hogs are the most natural virus reservoirs followed by chickens. They are naturally built to overproduce a kind of thick saturated fat called lard.

What is very disheartening about lard is that it is insoluble in water, by extension, in human tissue. Also, it depletes B vitamins. This means a person who cannot produce enzymes to break down lard and thoroughly process it will be susceptible to obesity.

Lard is the base substance of many products because it is an excellent emollient and lubricant. The products that have lard include: soaps, shaving cream and various cosmetic creams. Since the skin absorbs lard very easily, people who chew lard-based gums or use shaving cream or cosmetic creams that are made with lard will gain weight very easily or they will develop razor bumps or acne on the chin.

Hogs forage for food everywhere including dirt and mud; and they could also feed on feces. They are not affected by what they feed on because they produce enzymes that destroy E. coli and all kinds of bacteria. Unfortunately, their enzymes don't destroy cold and influenza viruses. This may explain why influenza always spreads from pigsties and from chicken coops.

Free-range hogs supply the unhealthiest meats. This is because when these hogs are hungry, they will feed on anything in their path. Since nutrition entails the transfer of plant or animal tissue to human tissue, eating pork will also imply transferring whatever is in pork to the tissue of the person who is eating it. This transfer also includes lard.

The main problem with lard is that it blocks circulation, it depletes B vitamins and also, it obstructs fat metabolism. This is why people who consume lard tend to become obese and also, they tend to suffer from osteoarthritis. When lard was fed to laboratory animals, they had a short life span compared to those that were not fed this saturated fat.

Sequestered hogs do not feed on feces but they are fed animal drugs; and these drugs are in their tissue. Ham, hotdog and bacon come from hog. Ham is made from the hind leg of the hog and bacon is made from the hog's belly, shoulder and loin.

Chapter Eighteen
Fish

Methyl mercury in some fish causes brain damage and manic depression. This is because it depletes B vitamins and zinc. The best fish are those that excrete 90% of the antibiotics that are fed to them. Such fish are farmed.

Fish, as a source of flesh protein, is better than chicken, turkey, pork and beef except for people who are allergic to fish.

Fish is healthier than meat because it causes the release of the smallest amount of uric acid after digestion. This will translate to fewer gout problems. Secondly, a person who replenishes h/her stock of B vitamins, copper, zinc and manganese will produce enough enzymes. These enzymes will enable h/her to digest fish thoroughly. People who are allergic to fish are not producing the enzymes that help to digest fish protein and oil.

Eating scavenger fish especially catfish could be a health hazard. This is because catfish has an infinite capacity for absorbing and retaining dioxin. Dioxin causes cancer.

Tilapia is the kind of fish that has a very low tolerance for heavy metals. Since tilapias do their best to avoid areas that have heavy metals, they are among the healthiest fish to eat.

Fish that are in waters near paper mills have learned to adapt to dioxin toxicity. This is why it is not safe to eat those fish.

Fish that don't spawn and feed in polluted areas tend to absorb PCBs (polychlorinated biphenyls) and other heavy metals. Salmon spawns (dies after laying its eggs). This is why most of salmon are free of heavy metals.

Reef dwelling fish such as red snapper and barracuda produce a poison called ciguatera. Ciguatera poisoning causes cramps, diarrhea, etc.

Fish that produce scombroid poison are: dolphin fish, tuna, bluefish, swordfish, mackerel and bonito. Scombroid poison forms in the fish's flesh. This often happens when the fishing boat's refrigeration breaks down due to thermostat malfunction. If this happens, all the catch will have to be thrown away.

The US Department of Agriculture has been making random inspection of fishing boats. This is to ensure that the refrigeration of commercial fishing boats is in good running condition.

Sardine is the best supplier of purine. Tilapia has the lowest concentration of heavy metals and salmon spawns and anchovies supply purine. These are the reasons that make eating tilapia, salmon, anchovies and sardine a very healthy habit.

I don't recommend eating raw fish for the following reasons. Raw trout and raw salmon have a fluke called troglorema salmincola. Its toxin prevents muscle cells from dividing. This inhibition could make a person susceptible to muscular dystrophy. Trout and salmon should always be cooked.

Also, fish that feed on plankton are very unhealthy. This is because plankton releases a neurotoxin called saxotoxin. Certain dinoflagellates produce this neurotoxin. How can a person know whether a particular fish fed on plankton or not? This is impossible to determine.

Finally, when the synchrometer is used on freshly caught fish, many fish test positive for marine tapeworms. This suggests that raw fish eaters could be infested with marine tapeworms. These tapeworms are well known for causing gas.

Japanese have the highest rate of stomach ulcer and stomach cancer. This could be the direct consequence of a tradition of eating raw fish whose saxotoxin also deplete B vitamins, oxygen and oxidase from the cells.

CHAPTER NINETEEN
WOMEN'S HEALTH

FEMALES EASILY DEPLETE IRON, ESTROGEN AND PROGESTERONE because of menstruation. Then, those who take birth control pills will deplete them faster. Finally, women who eat drugged meat will deplete their female sex hormones the fastest.

Why is a woman always experiencing hormonal imbalance and its devastating consequences? The reason is, after depleting raw materials during menstruation, she does not replace them.

After menstruating for only two years (age 13 to 15), a young girl may begin to experience menstrual cramps. This is because her estrogen level is too low. If she does not replenish her depleted stock of nutrients, she may experience breast problems sooner or later.

The seed for breast cancer in adulthood, abscess in the breast, pain in the breast, lactation problems and tumor or cyst in the breast or in the ovaries is planted very early in a woman's life.

Besides being humans, women have other issues that affect their health. These are: birth control pills, tubal ligation, estrogen replacement therapy (HRT) and hysterectomy. Then, abortion or miscarriage could cause chronic additional health problems.

All women are already plagued by chronic nutrient deficiencies; and the above-mentioned procedures and aids will make a complicated situation worse especially if women don't get the right advice as teenagers or as young adults.

Menstruation is by itself an iron drainer; and to get enough iron into the cells is not easy. Iron could be in the woman's blood but it will not diffuse into her cells if she is not producing PCM (protein carrier molecule). How does a woman produce PCM?

She will need copper in order to produce PCM but copper from food will not diffuse into her cells if she is also eating foods that have zinc. Then, zinc will not diffuse into her cells if she consumes a diet of insoluble fiber several times a week.

Why do women who think they are doing everything right still suffer from nutrient deficiencies? It is because they have not been informed that nutrients could be in the blood but they will diffuse into the cells only under certain conditions. Some of these conditions are what I just mentioned i.e. PCMs must be present and soluble fiber, not insoluble fiber must be consumed.

A woman who does not know how to replenish iron will be chronically anemic. Anemia in the brain is called cerebral anemia. Symptoms of cerebral anemia include: talking too much, cruelty, selfishness, jealousy and superficiality. They may appear to be typical of women. The truth is that all women don't engage in these behaviors. They are rather emblematic of cerebral anemia.

Symptoms of sub-clinical anemia compounded by hormonal imbalance include: heavy menses, prolonged menses, scanty menses and having a period again two weeks later.

Every form of contraceptive depletes zinc from the woman's body. Zinc is important for preventing inflammations. This is because cells add zinc to glutathione in order to produce GTP (glutathione peroxidase), a first class inflammation inhibitor. What is the difference between inflammation and pain?

Biochemical reactions that occur in the tissues produce tough debris. This debris will jam tissue. As a result, the circulation of endorphins (natural painkillers) will be impaired. This will cause pain. It is the absence of GTP that will make the cells to over-produce leukotrienes. Then, it is leukotrienes that will cause an inflammation where tissue will swell. If the swollen area does not have painkillers, it will become painful.

A pregnant woman who does not take the right kind of zinc daily for two weeks prior to delivery will find pain so unbearable that she will need epidural shot for some relief. Many women lost feelings in their arm or feet shortly after getting this shot.

Does it make sense to take an analgesic (man-made painkiller)? No, it does not. In order to be painless, a person should 1) supply the right kind of zinc to her body every other day and 2) abstain from consuming insoluble fiber.

The cells will take their time to produce SOD (superoxide dismutase) so that pain no longer occurs. If a woman eats a high fiber diet several times a week, zinc will be depleted. As a result, she will experience pain.

Pain is pain. Where it occurs is totally irrelevant. Women complain of pain in their kidney, waist, mid back, lower abdomen, stomach, knee, thigh, leg, eye, head, elbow, shoulder, hip, heel, toe, ear, teeth, jaw, throat, joints and so on and so forth. Again, pain occurs only where endorphins are absent. Taking a drug or smoking marijuana to treat pain is absolutely not the right way to address the root cause of pain.

Women tend to eat a high fiber diet because they are often constipated. This is not the right way to address the root cause of constipation. A special B vitamin called coenzyme A will help the colons to produce so much elastin that bowel movement will no longer be an issue.

Eating a diet of insoluble fiber several times a week or taking fiber supplements will deplete zinc. If a woman can't move her bowel it is because she lacks coenzyme A.

Colons produce elastin by mixing amyl acetate with B vitamins. Banana is the only acid fruit that has amyl acetate. Then, it is elastin that makes it possible for peristalsis (wavelike movement) to take place.

The natural bacteria in our colons are always producing a small amount of B vitamins, not for the whole body but just to produce elastin and to prevent pernicious anemia. A woman who takes antibiotics will wipe out the natural bacteria from her colons. Any woman who wants to be healthy should steer clear of antibiotics.

Will taking acidophilus replenish the depleted stock of natural bacteria? Not necessarily. There are about 30 different strains of natural bacteria in the colons. Acidophilus produces only one strain of bacterium. If the strain that produces vitamin B12 is not in the colons, the woman will be deficient in B12. The prolonged absence of B12 will predispose her to pernicious anemia.

Mastitis (inflammation of the breast), ovaritis (inflammation of the ovaries), metritis (inflammation of the uterus), cervicitis (inflammation of the cervix), endometriosis (inflammation of the endometrium) cephalgia (headaches), sarcoidosis etc. occur only in women whose zinc level is too low.

Sugar and hormonal imbalances cause fibroids, cysts, polyps or tumors. Sugar imbalance will deplete estrogen. This will offset the estrogen-progesterone ratio in a woman or the estrogen testosterone ratio in a man. This is why whenever I am treating a man or a woman I will also be correcting sugar and hormonal imbalances.

This book gives the kind of advice that will be of great value to many health conscious females. In so doing, it could stop them from making mistakes that will ruin their health in the future.

Every young girl must decongest her cells, nourish them properly and maintain sugar and hormonal balance at all times.

Men don't conceive. Women do. Since this is the case, every woman should know a symptometrist. The reason is, only symptometrists decongest cells, nourish them properly and maintain sugar and hormonal balance. These actions help a young girl to have monthly symptom-less menses.

If a woman continues to have symptom-less menses, she will never have a fertility problem, she will never suffer a miscarriage, never experience breast problems, emotional and mental problems and so on and so forth. If she conceives, symptometry will offer pregnancy management and after-birth care.

Is it my objective to produce a perfect woman and to raise her hope to the sky? No, this is not my objective. I am just affirming what symptometry can do for every woman on this planet. If I don't put in writing what symptometry can accomplish, nobody will do it for symptometry. Many women are healthier now thanks to symptometry.

There are four ways in which young women ruin their health. These are:

1) They do not decongest their cells
2) They do not nourish their cells properly
3) They do not maintain sugar and hormonal balance and
4) They use forms of contraceptives other than condom

Many young women start using contraceptives around age 16 without knowing the side effects of estrogen contraceptives, progestin contraceptives and combination contraceptives.

First of all, no contraceptive is 100% effective or safe. Secondly, striking the right balance between an occasional intercourse and getting an education and building a career is not easy for most women.

Nutrients do correct hormonal imbalance 70% of the time. Then, desired intercourse does the rest. A woman could take all the supplements she wants but if she does not have desired intercourse to satisfy the 30% of her hormonal needs, she will have emotional problems. Unfortunately, if she exceeds this 30%, she could become addicted to sex. Women who exceed their 30% tend to become either sexually promiscuous or they will suffer from nymphomania (uncontrollable sexual appetite).

A young woman must have occasional intimacy because it is her natural way of regulating hormonal balance. If she can't use intimacy to regulate 30% of her hormonal balance, she could be snappy, cranky, disrespectful, rebellious, mischievous, irritable, etc. There is no substitute for intercourse.

Why am I am discussing this issue? I am discussing it because most men don't understand women. Abstinence works only up to a point. If all men understood women, there will be peace on earth.

Peace is not found in church, in a mosque, synagogue, at a Heads of State summit, etc. It is found in a good relationship where hormonal needs are met. Good relationship is transformational and multi-dimensional.

Unfortunately, it is nutrient deficiencies that will result in promiscuity after an occasional intimacy and to sexually transmitted diseases (STD).

If a woman is infected with STD, how is she going to treat it? If she resorts to drug treatment, the bacteria will be destroyed but, according to microbiology, their toxin will remain in her system indefinitely; and this could cause tissue damage and sometimes infertility.

In order to have occasional intimacy without the risk of getting pregnant, I recommend that chemical contraceptive not be used. A means that will prevent the sperm from fusing with the egg is preferable. Condom prevents this fusion. Chemical contraceptives that have progestin will ruin a woman's health.

RU 486 and other pills are oral chemical contraceptives. Norplant, tubal ligation and IUD (intrauterine device) are other forms of quasi-chemical contraceptives.

Intrauterine device is a T-shaped piece of plastic that is placed inside the uterus. It either contains copper or man-made progesterone called progestin. It works by reducing the sperm's motility or by killing it.

Copper and man-made progesterone (progestin) will keep changing the lining of the uterus so that in case fertilization accidentally occurs, implantation of the blastocyst in the uterus will be impossible.

It is the constant changing of the lining of the uterus that could predispose a woman to endometriosis, to endometrial cancer or to uterine cancer. These diseases constitute one of the side effects of IUD.

Norplant is the name of the system that produces a long-term progestin-releasing contraceptive called *levonorgestrel*. It must be removed or replaced every five years. However, if the woman who has it is experiencing 1) pain or inflammation of the vein (phlebitis) 2) blood spitting due to blood clots in her lungs or 3) jaundice, the device will have to be removed without further delay.

Every contraceptive regardless of its name must deplete essential nutrients from the woman before it will be effective 80 to 90% of the time.

If copper, vitamin K and B vitamins are depleted, heavy menstrual bleeding will occur. If vitamin C and copper are depleted, chronic vaginal discharge will occur. If thiamine is depleted, the woman will not be able to metabolize sugar and also, she could experience severe menstrual cramps.

Furthermore, if riboflavin is depleted, the woman will not be able to cope with stress, she will be sensitive to many antibiotics, or she could develop bruxism (grinding of teeth), adult-onset epilepsy, multiple sclerosis or hypoglycemia.

If niacin is depleted, her estrogen and progesterone levels will be very low all the time, her blood could be full of toxins (toxemia), she could develop high blood pressure, diabetes mellitus, high cholesterol, high triglycerides, neurosis, psychosis, ulcers, skin disorders, bad breath, dizziness, chronic constipation or diarrhea.

When a woman seeks my expertise on certain health issues the first question I ask is "are you on some kind of birth control?" The second question depending on her age and on the number of children she has is "have you tied your tubes?" Then, if she is more than 50 years old I will enquire about her treatment with HRT.

The type of progestin, the level of estrogen in her body and the dose of progestin in the birth control pill will give a clue about the duration or the intensity of the woman's headaches; migraine, depression, severe pain in the left or right ovaries and pain in the calf. Ovaritis is the most common side effect of contraceptives.

Many women on birth control pills tend to suffer from all kinds of breast problems and from PID (pelvic inflammatory disease).

In order to cause the above-mentioned ailments, progestin and synthetic estrogen must be depleting B vitamins, zinc and GTP (glutathione peroxidase) on a daily basis. This is because B vitamins and zinc are central to the production of endorphins (natural painkillers); and B vitamins are important for the production of serotonin (for mood regulation).

Prescribing a painkiller for headache or for migraine or a drug for depression when a woman is on birth control pills is an exercise in total futility. It will amount to symptom treatment.

Before providing root cause treatment, a symptometrist will advise the woman to stop taking the pill and to use condom instead. This will minimize the depletion of her B vitamins and zinc. Cell decongestion will follow, B vitamins and the right zinc and chromium will be supplied to her cells at a certain frequency and rhythm. This will finally correct her sugar imbalance.

If a woman had her tubes tied and she has unprotected intercourse, she could become pregnant. Most of the pregnancies that occur under these circumstances result in ectopic pregnancies.

Chronic insomnia, runaway hypertension, very irregular menstruation and un-refreshed sleep are the most common complaints of women who underwent tubal ligation or hysterectomy. Such procedures disturb the natural pattern of blood flow in the pelvis and to the brain. This will in turn disrupt the functioning of the endocrine system.

Women have hysterectomy because they are tired of dealing with uterus-related health problems especially fibroids and uterine cyst.

The irony of the whole situation is that after hysterectomy has been performed, women usually realize that they will have to deal with a new set of problems. These include weight gain, unexplained chronic pain in the pelvis, insomnia, fatigue, constipation and symptoms of early menopause even though the ovaries have not been removed.

Why have hysterectomy when symptometry decompresses fibroids and cures every uterine disease? Life after hysterectomy could be very rocky. A surgical error that ends up damaging an internal organ during hysterectomy will certainly cause additional health problems for the woman.

Tubal ligation will obstruct circulation in the woman's pelvis. This will in turn offset her hormonal balance. Nothing works right in a woman whose hormones are out of balance.

She could be moody, irritable, impatient or depressed; or she could lose interest in intimacy or be indifferent to many issues. This could cause additional friction in an already fragile relationship.

Surgery to untie the tubes often causes a lot of tissue damage; and tissue damage will cause additional health problems.

Going off the pill should be done in a gradual manner so that as the intake frequency of the pill is being reduced, the intake frequency of B vitamins and other nutrients will be increased.

Estrogen replacement therapy (HRT) is the most controversial of all the procedures a woman undergoes. First of all, why is the woman's estrogen being replaced? If contraceptives had not depleted her estrogen, her estrogen level would have been normal. This scenario is similar to setting a house on fire and then, turning around to put out the fire and be hailed as a hero. If the house had not been set on fire, there wouldn't have been the need to put out the fire.

The following are the side effects of all contraceptives whether the woman is still using one of them or she stopped using them a few years back:

- Prolonged menses lasting 8 days or more
- Spotting (bleeding between periods)
- Menses occur every two weeks
- Heavy menses. Menses of anemic women will be heavier
- Absence of menses for three to four months without being pregnant. Then, suddenly, menstruation starts again. This could also cause unintended pregnancy
- Scanty menses lasting only a day or two
- Nausea
- Vomiting
- Anxiety attacks
- Headaches
- Migraine
- Dizziness

- Acne
- Weight gain
- Alopecia (scalp hair loss)
- Vaginitis (inflammation of the vagina)
- Chronic vaginal itch
- Cervicitis (inflammation of the cervix)
- Cervical cancer
- Breast discharge i.e. breast milk is flowing even though the woman is neither pregnant nor breastfeeding
- Mastalgia (severe breast pain)
- Hirsutism or hypertrichosis (woman develops facial hair, a lot of hair on her legs, arms, etc.)

Women who are on IUD or used to be on UID tend to experience one or several of the following:

- Weight gain
- Asthemia (fatigue/weakness)
- Severe cramps in the toes, legs, calf, fingers etc.
- Depression
- Breast cancer
- Myocardial infarction
- Urticaria (skin rash)
- Visual disturbance
- Pulmonary embolism (blood clot in the lung)
- Deep vein thrombosis (blood clot in the vein)
- Stroke
- Ectopic pregnancy
- Gallstones
- Gallbladder disease
- Hypertension
- Ovarian cysts
- Phlebitis (inflamed vein)

Women who use combination oral contraceptives (drugs that release man-made estrogen and progestin) tend to experience one or several of the following:

- Herpes due to change of skin pH (acid/alkali ratio). The skin is acidic with a pH of 6.2 just like that of urine. Some contraceptives and bath soaps make the skin too alkaline. Thus, making it a soft target for herpes simplex
- Retinal vascular lesion
- Retinal thrombosis (blood clot in the retina)
- Hepatic adenomas (liver tumors)

- Cervical intraepithelial neoplasia (invasive cervical cancer)
- Sugar imbalance
- Fluid imbalance resulting in fluid retention. Examples of fluid retention include: bags under the eyes, swollen eyelids, swollen legs and ankles or swollen knee
- Diabetes mellitus
- Stroke
- Morbid obesity where the woman could balloon up to 600 pounds. A woman who is on the pill and eats drugged meat such as drugged chicken, beef, etc. may not be able to control her weight because of sulfamethazine
- Myocardial infarction

It should be noted that women who are on the pill or have IUD and smoke, are ten times more likely to suffer from myocardial infarction (heart attack) than women who don't.

The reason myocardial infarction is more common in women who smoke is, carbon monoxide in cigarette smoke regardless of whether it is acidic or alkaline, will damage the splanchnic and vascular nerves of the capillaries in the heart. If these capillaries collapse as a result of this action, blood will stop flowing to a segment of the heart.

When a woman is sick, the root cause of her ailment must be determined and cleared so that her health can be restored at the cellular and tissue levels. Writing a prescription, doing case taking and repertorization and recommending herbs will never address the root cause of a woman's problems.

Nothing in a woman is a mystery. If she is sick it is because 1) she never decongested her cells or replenished her stock of nutrients 2) there is something in her system that keeps depleting essential nutrients and 3) nutrients that are being depleted by pharmaceutical drugs including antibiotics and contraceptives are not being replaced.

For instance, when a woman is losing her hair she tends to blame hair shampoo or her perm for this problem. In a woman, hair loss is the result of the effect of alkaline shampoo and the current or past use of contraceptives.

Weight gain is the direct result of sugar imbalance. This imbalance may cause poor fat metabolism. Contraceptives also cause sugar imbalance by depleting chromium.

Women are not aware that man-made estrogen, horse estrogen called premarin and progestin disrupt sugar metabolism in order to cause weight gain.

Will taking a multivitamin solve a woman's health problems? No, it won't. All women who are still sick despite taking multivitamins can attest to this fact.

Human cells are very well organized. For this reason, if a woman wants to replenish her stock of nutrients she must do so sequentially and rhythmically.

CHAPTER TWENTY
SALT

BLOOD HAS TO BE MARGINALLY ALKALINE BECAUSE IT CARRIES salt, a nuclear reactor. It is called a nuclear reactor because it causes a reaction in the nucleus of the cell as well as in blood.

Without salt, biochemical reactions would grind to a halt. It is biochemical reactions that facilitate the production of raw materials for cell division and for regular tissue production.

Plant salt is not human salt. Therefore, people who don't add salt to their food on the fire because the plants they are cooking have salt are making a big mistake.

Humans get their salt from rocks or from the sea. This salt is concentrated. Plant salt is too diluted just as its calcium; phosphorus, potassium, etc. are too diluted for human cells.

Furthermore, cooking makes plant salt to disappear and also it makes the food tasteless. Tasteless food does not put the taste buds to work. If the fibers in the nerves of the taste buds are not used daily, they will cease to function. As a result, the person will lose h/her sense of taste.

Sodium is indispensable to nerve function. The nerves run the human body. Therefore, a person who excludes salt from h/her diet will experience nerve disorders. Sooner or later, h/her heart will become weak; h/her sphincters, heart valves, ligaments, tendons and cartilage, etc. will become so weak that s/he could suffer from palpitation, incontinence, etc. No person who is on sodium-restricted diet is healthy.

52

Does eating salt cause hypertension? The answer is an emphatic no. If this were true, everybody on this planet who eats salt would suffer from hypertension. It is injury to the vagus nerve by calcium poisoning or by salicylate poisoning that causes hypertension. Excess calcium and salicylates will deplete phenylalanine that the vagus nerve uses to regulate blood pressure.

I know many people who like to eat very salty food but they don't have high blood pressure. The reason they don't have high blood pressure is they eat foods that keep supplying the amino acid called phenylalanine to their vagus nerve. They may not know this scientific reason but a symptometrist knows it.

Chapter Twenty-one
Sugars and Sweeteners

THERE ARE DIFFERENT KINDS OF SWEETENERS. A PRODUCT THAT is 300 to 600 times sweeter than table sugar has a different technical name. It is called a sweetener. The term "sugar" only applies to succharose that is also known as sucrose (white sugar).

Lactose, fructose, dextrose, sucrose and maltose are natural sugars. Animals produce lactose and plants produce fructose, dextrose, etc. Natural sugars are considered to be harmless.

The sweeteners are: high fructose corn syrup, low fructose corn syrup, sucralose, aspartame and saccharin as well as the 16 other kinds of sucrose-based sweeteners.

The difference in the name comes from the fact that a product that a chemist made in a laboratory is no longer considered to be sugar. In other words, it is not natural.

Splenda that is best known as sucralose was made in a laboratory. It is 600 times sweeter than sugar. In April 1998, the FDA (Food and Drug Administration) approved its use in all diet drinks, baked goods, tabletops, confections, desserts and fruit spreads.

If a person who is overweight drinks diet coke because it has fewer calories, s/he will only lose a few pounds. This is because sucralose will continue to block fat metabolism by causing sugar imbalance.

The calorie count is just a gimmick. Eating too many calories does not cause obesity. It is rather sweeteners, which block the metabolism of fat, and eating drugged meat that make a person to gain weight unnecessarily.

Saccharin is 300 times sweeter than sugar. In animals, it is a carcinogen. Unfortunately, if a person has cancer it would be very difficult to connect saccharin to h/her disease. Some diet sodas also have saccharin. Rats that were fed saccharin developed bladder tumors.

Aspartame is popularly known as NutraSweet. It is 200 times sweeter than sugar. It has been linked to brain tumors. In 1981, the FDA approved its use in breath mints, chewing gums, fruit juices, instant coffee, instant tea, ready-to-serve non-alcoholic beverages, malt drinks, fruit concentrates, syrups, icings for pre-cooked baked goods, frostings, toppings, fillings and glazes.

Aspartame lowers the acidity of urine and it makes the bladder to become very susceptible to chronic infections and to inflammation. Again, aspartame causes brain tumor.

Beginning of sugar-related diseases

According to historical accounts, "the reed which gives honey without the bees" grew in the ancient islands of Polynesia. Over 1,000 islands formed Polynesia. Then, people in the neighboring land mass started cultivating "the reed". Finally, Indians also started cultivating it. The original Indian land was very vast. Unfortunately, much of it was lost to conquerors.

In 510 B.C., the forces of Emperor Darius of Persia invaded India and they discovered that the natives were using sugar that they had extracted from sugar cane.

Emperor Darius took over the sugar enterprise. For centuries, Persia became very rich from the sugar trade, which they called "sweet spices". This wealth made them to engage in Arab expansionism in order to spread Islam. Wherever they conquered they established sugar plantation and production. This included North Africa and Spain.

It was the Crusades of the 11th century that introduced the Spaniards to sugar and how to cultivate it. The Spanish conquistadors who invaded Central and South America introduced sugar cane cultivation to the natives.

Equally, in 1493, Christopher Columbus took some sugar canes with him and after landing on different Caribbean islands his crew taught the natives how to cultivate sugar cane. This was how the Western world was introduced to sucrose in the sixteenth century.

As a matter of record, before the conquistadors landed in South America, the native South Americans already had their natural plant sugar that they had been using for over a thousand years. It is now called stevia.

Unfortunately, stevia produced such a small amount of sugar after processing that the conquistadors were not interested in it. They wanted a product that could be produced in very large quantities so that they would help their government back home to make more money. This was why they preferred the cultivation of sugar cane to that of stevia. With sugar cane and cotton cultivation came the slave trade.

By 1750 there were 120 sugar refineries operating in Great Britain. According to estimates, they collectively produced 30,000 tons of sugar a year. Sugar generated so much tax revenue for the British and other European governments that it was dubbed "the white gold".

Sugar beet was identified as a source of sugar much later in 1747. Sugar was such a sweet and much sought after item that, culinary experts and food manufacturers went after it wherever they could find it. What they did not know was that too much sugar makes it impossible for the body to process it properly.

Because excess sugar depletes thiamine and chromium from the body, it makes it impossible for the pancreas to produce enough insulin, the adrenal gland to produce enough cortisol and the liver to produce enough enzymes to convert glucose to glucagon. As a result, the excess glucose that circulates in blood becomes very destructive to the tissues especially to the nerves. Moreover, white blood cells can't function properly when there is too much glucose in blood.

Sugar-related diseases did not start in the nineteenth century. It is believed to have started as a result of the use of sugar in Asia and this was before the advent of the Roman Empire.

Little is known about the Polynesians except that they were seafarers, they built boats before Archimedes formulated his buoyancy principle and they invented the process for extracting sugar from sugar cane.

Polynesians and other Asians who consumed sugar had cancer. This was before the Romans got to know that there was a disease called cancer. Claudius Galen, originator of allopathy, named the disease cancer because to him, it looked like crab's feet (karkinos). What was he really looking at?

Today, cancer treatment has become a pot of gold for the pharmaceutical industry. Cancer is a totally curable and preventable disease. Tumors are also preventable.

A person, who knows that it is the body's inability to properly metabolize sugar and produce the enzyme called oxidase, will be able to cure or prevent cancer. Why can't the body metabolize sugar? It is because chromium and thiamine have never been supplied to it in years.

Why is it that the first advice a cancer patient gets is s/he should avoid eating strong sugar? The answer is cancer feeds off sugar. It is poor sugar metabolism that causes cancers and ulcers.

Cancer may start as a tumor but it will create countless ulcers and lesions in its victim before s/he dies. Also, it will make the person to lose appetite. If a person can't produce protein because s/he is not eating enough food, s/he will be emaciated. Every cancer patient is emaciated before s/he dies.

For people who are not aware, strong sugars (sweeteners) are the world's number one nutrient depleting agents. They even prevent fats from being processed. This will make a person either skinny or overweight.

Will avoiding eating sugar prevent sugar-caused diseases? No, it won't. A person who avoids eating sugar will get sugar-caused diseases just as a person who eats a lot of it.

A lot of glucose in blood will deplete chromium just as sweeteners in foods will deplete chromium and thiamin. This is why, whether a person abstains from eating sugar or not, s/he will still suffer from chromium and thiamin deficiencies. This will in turn translate to sugar imbalance.

The sugar-caused diseases or the health problems that are caused by sugar imbalance are as follows:

- High blood pressure because the vagus nerve has been injured due to the chronic absence of phenylalanine
- Infertility because a woman who can't metabolize sugar can't support life in the womb. Sugar is the backbone of DNA.
- Pain because these two nutrients are not available for the cells to produce endorphins.
- Diabetes mellitus because the pancreas, the adrenal gland and the liver have been denied phenylalanine, chromium and thiamin for years.
- Chronic infections because the T cells need NADP, zinc, manganese, chromium and thiamin to produce hydrogen peroxide and

bacteriocin. Without these nutrients, they will stay aloof and allow the pathogens to damage the tissues
- Low white blood cell count
- Hyperactivity
- Hypoglycemia
- Sugar craving
- Fatigue or lethargy
- All cancers
- Low immunity
- Eczema
- Psoriasis
- Depression
- Eating disorders including anorexia and bulimia
- Forgetfulness
- Anxiety attacks
- Irritability
- Violent temper
- Cataract
- Panic attacks
- Inability to concentrate or lack of focus
- Absentmindedness
- Attention deficit disorder
- Forgetfulness
- Lack of confidence
- Lack of motivation
- Lack of enthusiasm
- Emotional imbalance
- Obesity
- Gum disease
- High cholesterol
- Aggressive behavior and
- Type A personality
- Acne
- High triglycerides
- Inability to thoroughly metabolize fats and oils

A person is a sugar-dependent biological entity. This is why if s/he can't process sugar s/he can't be healthy.

Chapter Twenty-two
Nutrition, The Double Edged Sword

Nutrition is a double-edged sword. This is because no matter what we eat, we will always end up sick unless we prevent the sickness. In other words, if we eat, in the short run, we will be healthy but in the long run we will have an acute symptom. If we treat this acute symptom with a mismatch, it will turn into a chronic symptom. Let me explain this paradox.

Whatever we eat will be broken down during digestion that begins in the mouth. Digestion will release the food constituents that will then circulate to the small intestine. After assimilating the nutrients, the small intestine will circulate them to the liver. The liver will store and ration the nutrients to the cells that need them. This is what happens in theory. In practice, many cells will never get what they need. Here is why.

Vanadium and molybdenum are two elements that our cells don't need. Since our cells don't need them, they will have nowhere else to go. This is why they will become nutrient blockers until many cells have produced enough enzymes to liquefy them. If we eat foods that have nutrients and nutrient blockers, the nutrient blockers will prevent the nutrients from getting into our cells. As a result, our cells will be impoverished.

People can eat all they want and yet they will not be able to lose weight or they will remain skinny. People are anorexic or bulimic because the foods they are consuming have nutrient blockers. Then, people have ulcers, lesions or fractures that can't heal because they are consuming nutrient blockers.

Vanadium in some of the following foods will prevent almost every nutrient from getting into the cells: corn, green beans, peanut oil, carrots, cabbage, radishes, buckwheat, soybeans, oats, parsley, olive oil, apples, mil-

DR. MAXWELL NARTEY, DHM, NHD

let, mushrooms, shellfish, black pepper, beets, plums, lettuce and whole wheat.

Molybdenum is not one of the 26 minerals like sodium, calcium, magnesium, sulfur, silicon, phosphorus, etc. that are indispensable to human existence. In other words, plants need molybdenum but humans don't need it. Whatever the cells don't need will become a nutrient blocker until it is eliminated.

The items that have molybdenum are: lentil, split peas, cauliflower, corn, green peas, green beans, rye bread, barley, carrots, barley, whole wheat bread, potatoes, raw onions, cantaloupe, peanuts, brewer's yeast, wheat germ, spinach, brown rice, garlic, oats, butter, cabbage, strawberries, raisins and apricot.

Foods that have molybdenum, vanadium or wax may be someone's favorite but since molybdenum is a nutrient blocker it is recommended that such foods be eaten once a week so that cells produce enough enzymes to eliminate what they don't need. At least cells can eliminate nutrient blockers from food after 5 days or after a week but there are nutrient blockers that they can't eliminate unless they have been ionized.

Calculus, calcareous deposits, tophus and gouty deposits are the nutrient blockers that our cells cannot eliminate. How did each of these blockages form?

Apples, peaches, pears, etc. that do not come directly from farms have been waxed. Therefore, a person who does not peel off the skin of fruits before juicing or eating them will also ingest wax. Wax is a nutrient blocker.

About 75 trillion cells make up the human body. Out of this number, about 6 million of them will have to breakdown every twelve hours so that new cells can be produced. Red blood cells must break down after 120 days. After deconstruction, the entire structure of the cell turns into calculus. The residues of calcium will turn into calcareous deposits. After deconstruction, DNA will turn into uric acid. Then, after a while, uric acid will harden to form gouty deposits. Gout releases sodium urate. This will harden to form tophus.

We have an excretory system. Unfortunately, this excretory system does not eliminate gout, tophus, calcareous deposits and calculus from our body. It only eliminates sweat, urine, carbon dioxide and feces. What makes our problem worse is that sodium in our blood will react with the residue of every nutrient to produce either soft or tough debris.

For instance, after chewing the hard shell of crustaceans (lobster, shrimp, crab, etc.), the chewed mass will react with sodium in blood to produce tough debris. Others that will produce tough debris include: sucrose, sucralose, aspartame, saccharin, oxalates in spinach; beans, boiled eggs, baking soda, indigestible items, gluten, nuts, seeds, cucumber, millet, rye, barley, red meat and wheat.

After digestion, cells will produce enzymes to liquefy debris. Incidentally, soft debris will be liquefied faster than tough debris. If tough debris remains un-liquefied for weeks, it will begin to jam the cells of the kidneys and bladder. As a result, incontinence and kidney disease could occur. Sometimes, tough debris could jam the cells in other segments of the body.

Nephritis and glomerulo-nephritis (Bright's disease) are classic examples of kidney diseases. Symptoms of kidney congestion include: high level of creatinine, protein in urine, glucose in urine, smelly urine, delayed urination, inability to urinate, very scanty urine, epithelium in urine, mucus or oil in urine, brown color of urine, sediment in urine and gold color of urine.

Therefore, the kind of food a person eats is very important. A person who wants to have healthy bladder and kidneys should eat foods that produce soft debris more often. These foods include: lactose-free, dairy-free and unsweetened milk, pasta, fish, banana, avocado, certain vegetables and rice.

A person can eat selectively but if s/he does not sanitize h/her circulatory and lymphatic systems by removing tophus, gout, calcareous deposits and calculus, chances are that s/he will not be healthy sexually, physically, organically, mentally, metabolically, emotionally or systemically. This is because nutrients will not be able to diffuse into h/her brain cells, nerve cells, dental cells, bone cells, muscle cells, skin cells, ligament cells, cartilage cells, tendon cells, etc.

If nutrients are not diffusing into nerve cells, numbness or pain will occur. If nutrients are not diffusing into muscle cells, muscular dystrophy or emaciation will occur. If nutrients are not diffusing into the bone cells of the vertebrae, multiple sclerosis may occur or the spine could be curved. If nutrients are not diffusing into the internal organs, kidney disease, liver disease, spleen disease, heart disease, lung disease, brain disease, bowel disease, gallbladder disease, etc. could occur.

People have joint disease because nutrients are not diffusing into the cells of the ligaments, cartilage, tendons and synovial membrane that form their joints. People have gum disease, toothache, dental cavities, bone cancer or bone pain because nutrients are not diffusing into the cells of the tooth, gum or bone. Muscles are sore or people bruise easily because nutrients are not diffusing into their muscle fibers.

The brain has several segments. The segments that are not receiving nourishment because of blockages will begin to produce mental or emotional symptoms. Forgetfulness; propensity for violence, irritability, indifference, academic dullness, stealing, addictions, etc. occur because blockages have not been removed from specific brain cells. All endocrinal disorders occur because the glands are congested and malnourished.

The liver has 15 segments. The segment that is congested will cause specific symptoms. The small intestine has a segment that produces lactase, a segment that produces protein-splitting enzymes, etc. If a segment is congested, it will simply not function again. Breaking down physiological facts in this manner makes it easy to track down a symptom to its source in a congested gland, segment or organ.

Is medical diagnostics necessary? Yes, it is to some extent because it can help to detect tumors, aneurysm, organ enlargement, lesions, cancer, low T cell count, low iron, glucose in blood, fluid in the brain, fluid in the lungs, damaged heart valve, broken bones, abscesses, high PSA (prostate specific antigen) and a few other abnormalities.

The abnormalities that medical diagnosis detects, account for only 3 to 4% of medical cases. The root cause of the remaining 96 to 97% of ailments cannot be detected by medical diagnostics.

For instance, can medical diagnosis detect the cause of the following? Hallucination, delirium tremens, menstrual cramps, menstrual irregularities, intermittent heartbeat, migraine, insomnia, numbness, violent behavior, propensity to steal, propensity to kill, mischief, grinding of teeth, sleeping with the eyes half open, inability to close the mouth, ringing in the ear, hissing noise in the ear, macular degeneration, detached retina, curved spine, receding gum line, inability to open the eyes, palpitation, hearing one's own heartbeat, deformed nail, blue nail, brown urine and three thousand more of such abnormalities. No, it can't. However, breaking down physiological facts will lead a symptometrist directly to the root cause of these ailments.

Why do the abnormalities that medical devices detect occur? For instance, what causes fibroid tumors? What causes cancer? What causes an enlarged heart, an enlarged breast, a defective valve, an enlarged prostate, fluid in the lungs, fluid in the brain and so on and so forth?

The root cause of every complaint is a blockage that prevented oxygen, iron, calcium, potassium, sodium and other nutrients from getting into the cells; or a blockage that prevented wastes from leaving the cell. If food had not been digested and biochemical reactions had not taken place in the body, would these blockages in the form of calculus and deposits have formed? No, they wouldn't. What is my point?

The point I am making is that it is the process of digesting food and the thousands of biochemical reactions that ensue that cause blockages to form in order to ruin our health. Therefore, if a person places emphasis on good nutrition without sanitizing his systems and decongesting h/her cells, s/he will sooner or later suffer from one of the following: hair loss, dry skin, brittle bones, brittle nails, dry lips, pain in the ribs, lower back pain, pain in the tail bone, forgetfulness, painful joints, swollen joints, bleeding gums, dry hair, pain in the ear, etc. If oxygen does not get into some cells in a specific segment of h/her body, s/he will get cancer at that site.

Is cancer a mystery disease? No, it is not. It is the cells that have been deprived of oxygen for ten years or more that will be cancerous. A person can eat a balanced diet and take dietary supplements but if s/he does not producing oxidase and sucrase, one of h/her cells will become cancerous.

Nutrition is the greatest paradox of all time. If a person eats, s/he will produce blockages. As a result, s/he will be sick sooner or later. If s/he does not eat, s/he will produce ten times more blockages. As a result, s/he will die of starvation.

Therefore, placing emphasis on good nutrition; exercise and meditation will leave blockages in a person's body. Such a half-measured approach will make a person healthy on only two or three fronts out of seven. People who want to be healthy on all the seven fronts will definitely find the half-measure approach of nutrition unappealing.

The most suitable way to promote comprehensive health is to recommend that cells be decongested and that tissues should be nourished in such a way that a person will keep producing an enzyme surplus. This will remove calculi, calcareous deposits, gouty deposits, etc. from the glands, internal organs, skin, nails, hair follicles and shaft, epitheliums, bones, teeth, nerves, muscle fibers in different parts of the body especially the throat, valves, sphincters, eye lids, eye balls, lips, tongue, tonsils, etc.

Health should not be reduced to only one narrow component called physical health. The sex organ, the bones, the muscles, the sphincters, the valves, all the internal organs, tendons, nerves, ligaments, cartilage, metabolism, the mind, and emotions as well as the circulatory and lymphatic systems must also be healthy before a person can claim that s/he is healthy on all the seven fronts.

There is no such thing as being 40% healthy, 60% healthy or 80% healthy. Either a person is healthy on all the seven fronts or s/he is not. Either a person is alive or s/he is dead. This is because there is no such thing as being 50% alive.

No molecule can remove calculus and cellular debris from the cells. Botanical products, vitamins and pharmaceutical drugs are molecules. This is why they can't remove blockages from the cells in order to make a person healthy on all the seven fronts.

Only sub-atomic particles in specific homoeopathic particulates have proven to be capable of removing blockages from the cells. This is why only specific homoeopathic particulates cure cyanosis, stasis, numbness, tingling, hemorrhaging black blood, etc.

Unfortunately, the way homoeopathy is taught in homoeopathic schools leaves much to be desired. This is because the word "cell" is not even mentioned in the curriculum. Then, repertorization that is used to select homoeopathic remedies is the most archaic method in the history of medicine. Finally, homoeopathy teaches thirteenth century vitalism that has absolutely no place in modern scientific thinking. How then do homoeopathic remedies work?

To get the answer, one must visit symptometry, not homoeopathy. Homoeopathic particulates work through the scientific process called blockage ionization and fault line closure.

Blockages prevent healing and also, they prevent a person from being healthy on all the seven fronts. Blockages include wax, tophus, gouty deposits, calculus, cellular debris and calcareous deposits. Spasms cause the formation of fault lines in the body. These fault lines must be closed. If they are not closed, diseases such as asthma and epilepsy or symptoms such as cough and irregular heartbeat will be chronic.

Symptometry uses the affinity concept to select specific homoeopathic particulates. It is these particulates that will ionize blockages in target cells. As soon as the blockages are removed or the fault line is closed, nutrient diffusion and osmosis will resume, waste will flow out of the cells, cells will divide and healing will begin. Health on all the seven fronts depends on constant healing at the cellular level. Stay tuned for part two.

REFERENCES

- *A Consumer's Dictionary of Food Additives* by Ruth Winter, M.S. Copyright 1978, 1984, 1989, 1994, 1999, 2004. Published by Three Rivers Press, New York, New York

- *A Consumer's Dictionary of Cosmetic Ingredients* by Ruth Winter, M.S. Copyright 1978, 1984, 1989, 1994 1999. Published by Three Rivers Press, New York, New York

- *Encyclopedia of Nutritional Supplements* by Michael T. Murray, ND Copyright 1996. Published by Prima Publishing. P.O Box 1280BK, Rocklin, CA 95677

- Burton, G.W. Journal of nutrition, vol 119, page 109 1989

- Bendich A. Clinical nutrition, vol 7, page 113, 1988

- Gridley, DS et al, Nutrition research, vol 8, page 201, 1988

- *Poisons in your Food* by Ruth Winter M.S, published by Crown Publishers, Inc, 201 East 50th Street, New York, New York 10022 Copyright 1969, 1991

- *Healthy Living* by Linda Page, Ph. D, published by Healthy Living, Inc copyright August 2006

INDEX